The Mechanics of Love
Victoria Gatehouse

smith|doorstop

Published 2019 by
Smith|Doorstop Books
The Poetry Business
Campo House
54 Campo Lane
Sheffield S1 2EG

Copyright © Victoria Gatehouse 2019
All Rights Reserved

ISBN 978-1-912196-66-1

Designed and Typeset by Utter
Printed by Biddles Books

Smith|Doorstop Books are a member of Inpress:
www.inpressbooks.co.uk. Distributed by NBN International, Airport Business Centre, 10 Thornbury Road Plymouth PL6 7PP

The Poetry Business gratefully acknowledges the support
of Arts Council England.

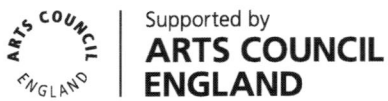

Contents

5	Inosculation
6	Ceiling
7	Poison, 1986
8	Sixth Form Science Technician
9	Walking the Boulevard
11	Shunkley
12	The Mechanics of Love
14	Fortune Teller Fish
15	Circuit
16	Naming Clouds
17	Pearl Daughter
18	Medusa Cuts Off Her Snakes
20	Victorian Housewives and The Art of Grief
21	Love Locks on the Pont des Arts
22	Indian Blue Peacocks For Sale
23	Pellets
24	Dogs' Balls
25	Poem for the Premier Inn
26	Web on the Wing Mirror
27	Cord
28	Side Effects
29	The Dog Who Played With His Shadow
30	Clearing
31	Acknowledgements

In memory of my grandmother, Elizabeth Collins

Inosculation

And this will be no perfect union
but one born of abrasion; two trees
grown close enough to graze, to chafe
as they shift in the wind, their bark worn thin,

rubbed down to the gleam of the cambium,
the raw lustre of vascular tissue.
This might be branch to branch or trunk
to trunk or even branch to trunk, a meld

of cells, a wound healed to a rise and shine.
Some call them marriage trees, some say these grafts
once fused and sealed, transmit disease
or claim the heartwood isn't touched, but once

I saw two beeches, interlocked,
initials scratched across the place they joined.

Ceiling

Mum asks which pattern
would I like on my ceiling;
all these 'artistic textures'
and a name for each one –

Stipple, tiny stalactites, dabbed on
with bristles; *Broken Leather*
involving a polythene bag.

I'm taken with the grooves
of *Fan* or *Shell*,
flowing on repeat
from a wide-toothed comb
but then *Swirl* draws me in

and he gets to work quickly,
the Artex man –
from the edge of his brush,
rhythms practiced and slick –

he's churning out whirlpools,
meringues whipped and set,
endless vortices
like the start of Dr Who,

spiral galaxies
that will never hold glow stars.

Poison, 1986

Back then you'd record
the Channel 4 breaks
intent on tracking her down –

vamp-nailed tamer
of black panthers,

her hands all you ever saw,
yet you could practically
inhale those base notes

through the screen – amber,
rosewood, musk, as she held up

the gleaming amethyst
glass-apple of a bottle.
Thirty seconds of decadence –

drenched in patchouli,
jasmine spice, plum-thick

wanting her scent, her life –
brazen dark-purple
dynamite, not your own

safe-sweet schoolgirl reek
of gym kit and Midget Gems.

Sixth Form Science Technician

The biology teacher wanted blood,
more than the usual finger-prick smear
for the microscopes. It was me she sent
on a two-bus journey to the abattoir.

Two weeks into the job and my days so far –
checking Bunsen valves, bottle-brushing
conical flasks, laying out spatulas
on asbestos mats, had not prepared me
for the man in his gore-stained apron,
gloved like a surgeon, that twist
of a smile as he took the empty jam jar,
closed a metal door in my face. No more

than thirty seconds and he handed it back,
slippery-lidded. Unexpected, the thick
warmth carried through glass, the dark
shift of particles inside. A bus caught,
and then another. Cooling in my lap,
that container of pigs' blood, sloshing
beneath its brown paper cover.

Fortune Teller Fish

> *Place the Fortune Teller Fish in your hand and its movements will indicate your future.*

In those days *Passion* was a total curl-up
willed into being by your teenage self,
a barely-there wafer of cellophane
turning over on your lifeline,
a Christmas cracker game
where you'd try and wriggle out
of side-lift *Fickle,* back-flip *False,*
the impassive red gleam of the *Dead One.*

A scientist now, you could explain
that whisper-thin strip as hygroscopic –
swelling or receding with the level
of moisture in the skin, a material so light
it shapeshifts on a breath, but lay
it on your palm, you'll find yourself wanting
to show you've still got it in you
to raise that *Independent* flag of a tail.

Walking the Boulevard

I remember kitten heels clipping tarmac
all the way down Lenton Boulevard,
a black patent handbag firm-gripped

and kids mincing behind
calling out *Tranny*, but he out-strode
even the late-for-lecture students,
turning every head as he passed –

the crooked crimson line of his lips,
that suggestion of dark growth
beneath American Tan tights,
the way his muscles strained
against beige corduroy seams.

Someone said he'd been seen
queening it at *The Birdcage* in stilettos
and a sequinned dress, but it wasn't true;
he was too slipshod for the nightclub scene –
jacket unstitched, Kirby grips dangling
from strands of his mid-brown wig.

Once, in the shelter for the Beeston bus
he pulled down the folding seat beside me,
unsnapped that black patent bag –

his fingers with their bitten and painted nails
all clumsy tenderness as he opened
a compact with a scalloped edge –

that shameless slick of blue
on lowered lids and a scent,
like dead flowers, rising

beneath the tang of his sweat.
All his late wife's things now his.

I can still see him, hunched
over that smudged and cracked mirror,
pressing her powder into the lines of his face.

The Mechanics of Love

It ticks me to sleep,
the titanium valve in your heart,

so close, my lips could press
a gleam down the horizontal scar

where they opened you up,
hooked cannulised veins

to the heart-lung machine.
This room of ours, all soft

darkness until a car passes;
in the place where curtains

don't quite meet, a spill
of light, making me think

of that imperfect seal,
how blood streaked back

from ventricle to atrium,
more turbulent with every year.

Now, the deep red
chambers of your heart, secured

against the leak and tonight,
every night, in that pause

between beats –
titanium, titanium,

for its strength, durability,
its resistance to corrosion,

for this love, for those two
shining leaflets

clicking in their frame,
hinging on it.

Shunkley

It was my mum's friend Sylvia
who gave us the word
which surfaced those rare nights
they went down the Lawnswood Arms

in response to a lurex motif
on a for-best blouse, the dusted-off
lustre of a marcasite brooch:
Jennifer you've got your shunkley on!

And it lingered, the word, to adorn
those first clubbing nights in Leeds –
sequinned dresses shimmering
beneath strobe-lights

before the all-in-black student days
when it revealed itself in a flash
of silver rings, the spark of a nose stud
because it won't be quietened,

this magpie need for a hint of bling –
a jewelled collar, a metallic cuff,
a tinsel halo for Christmas, a diaman*té*
pendant to lift that little black dress,

my gran on her ninetieth
propped up in a hospice bed,
fingers moving in slow wonder
across the cool facets

of a glass diamond necklace, glittering
hard above the morphine drip.

Circuit

Seven bars of galvanised steel, ideal for leaning on
to take in a field patched with nettle and docks,
a long view of moorland, copses of sycamore and ash,
and somewhere distant to all this, the motorway.

Horses, fetlock-deep in pale grass, raise heads
when my dog, eight-months and curious,
scrabbles across a slump in the stones.

I call him back, turn at the farmer's laugh.
It's switched off he says *but they don't know that*
and it takes a moment for my vision to snag
on frayed lengths of tape, threaded
through the plastic loops of insulator stakes.

These horses, who've ambled over to stand
soft-lashed at the gate (though I've nothing to give),
they'll no longer think beyond this field –
its tin bath of water, its buttercups, its circuit
of remembered pain. I leash the dog, walk on,
consider the boundaries of my own life,
which ones might not be live.

Naming Clouds

This morning I watched pale shreds
form a mezzanine above the reservoir,
thought back to the time we abandoned
the car, took the path across the moors,

the hum of the motorway
receding with each step until we found
the perfect place for a blanket
and afterwards, your hand in mine
as we slept, a glaze of heather at our backs.

Remember waking to a white-rag sky,
me re-tying windblown hair, that propensity
of yours to classify – *stratus fractus*.
I preferred *messenger clouds*.

Whatever you chose to call them,
we tasted rain long before
the vertical sweep across the moors,
that falling through of what lay above.

Pearl Daughter

And if I'm to dive, let it be like an Ama woman
in Ago Bay, bare backed and free
from the compressed weight of oxygen,
the skin around my eyes unmarked
by the seal of a shadow mask. Let me rise
before dawn, join the women who make
dockyards tilt and dip with bamboo flares,
hair bound by tenugi, long knives slipped
into fundoshi at their hips. And let my strong toes
propel me down to thirty feet and my lungs
become the lungs of the sea, bronchioles streaming
like weed, alveoli blown out to a coral-red bloom,
two minutes grace to gather sea urchins, lobsters,
to scrape alabone from rocks, and before I break
the surface, exhale that long slow whistle
to prevent the bends, let me haul up a bucketful
of oysters, just one pearl being enough to feed
a family for a week. And if I'm to bear a daughter,
let her swim before she can walk, let her hair
spread into a thousand salty whispers at her back,
let her pray to the glimmering eye of the shrine
for my safe return, and when she's twelve
or thirteen, body waking to the push and pull
of the tide, let her heed my warnings
of octopus lovers and sharks and I'll concede
the use of Neoprene. And if she follows her mother,
takes on the muscle and clout of the sea,
let her body be a twist of flame the ocean can't douse.

Medusa Cuts Off Her Snakes

They speak in tongues
    only I understand;
        consonants soft, uncoiling

    like temple prayers
and there were days
when I fed them tales

of my beauty, how I held
    the shine of waves
        the length of my spine,

    how men turned to look,
and look again.
It's the nights I dread,

the sea rolling in like a curse,
    the snakes whispering,
        mouths venom-slick,

    not letting me forget
Poseidon, in the temple –
all the force of the ocean

in him, his body hard
    as altar stone and afterwards
        the sting of salt in all the places

    he had been, the rage that grew
on me, scale-tight, a skin
that can't be shed.

At my feet, the swords of those
    who would turn from my stare.
        I lift a blade, cut deep, deeper,

        and it's hissing out of me
    all this pain, warm and easy
as a letting down of hair.

Victorian Housewives and The Art of Grief

My sister and I in our dark parlour,
weaving jewels from the hair of those we've lost –
feather-soft curls, stiff with homemade paste,
a cousin's plait, shining as it did in life,

this braiding and folding of sorrows,
painstaking formations of clouds, weeping-
willows, forget-me-nots, urns, enclosed
by white-enamel scrollwork, seed-pearl tears.

For each death, our black-edged year and a day,
the lick of the fire in carved jet beads, the ache
sealed into lockets and rings. We don't need
tea leaves to picture our husbands' oiled fringes

glued into keepsakes with our powdered locks,
displayed behind glass at our daughters' necks.

Love Locks on the Pont des Arts

Over forty tonnes of padlocks
swivelled and clicked into slots,
keys thrown over the edge to twist
bright and silver as fish in the Seine,
over seven hundred thousand names,
engraved and etched into alloys,
pen-knife scratched over brass,
scrawled across nickel with Tippex
or indelible ink, embellished
with acrylic kisses and nail-varnish hearts.
Myleen and David, Olly and Frank
Lolita and Si, Noya and Mark,
combinations forgotten or unknown,
secured with stainless steel tongues,
internal mechanisms of die-cast zinc,
by those who may or may not
be together still, but not here to see
their love locks hacked open
with bolt-cutters by men in hi-vis
and dumped into trucks so the grillwork
of the bridge, collapsed from the weight,
can be replaced with clear-panelled
Plexiglass. Now couples can gaze
through their own reflections,
imagine perhaps, that heap of keys
on the river's bed, the sleeping back
of some mythical creature,
a glint in its nearly-closed eye.

Indian Blue Peacocks For Sale

Just the sight of a feather in a peacock's tail ... makes me sick
– Charles Darwin, 1860

Held on red at the ring road lights
I see the advert scrawled on sawn-off chipboard
a mobile number and price (sixty-five quid)
and I'd quite like to ring and ask if that's for a chick
or a full-grown bird and do peacock breeders
like those who sell puppies   only let them go
to forever homes and wouldn't that be a farm
or even a country estate because didn't I read
that peacocks need space   more than can be found
in sunless back yards and aren't their turquoise
and bronze feathers too insistently luminous
to be trailed over tarmac   displayed against concrete
and how could this small litter-hurling sky
hold their magnificent evolution-defying weight
wouldn't plastic cartons splinter their proud beaks
but just supposing their shimmering throats didn't gag
on the remains of curry sauce and chips   pecked
from the astonished mouths of bins   imagine how
musters of them might dust-bathe in gutters   roost
on the cold shoulders of pylons   act out their quivering
deep-blue rituals in the piss-reek alleys of city estates
screech and signal from the bonnets of parked-up cars
and how Darwin would turn away   sickened
by the thought of females having the power to shape
these tails   not at all cock-a-hoop at having
to look again into all those raised eyes.

Pellets

This is the hour when she thinks of the field,
the unsteady embrace of dry-stone walls,
end-of-summer grasses, whispering
their untidy truths, the tooth-hole ruin

of that barn where she first found the pellets –
dark, neat parcels of feathers and fur,
the pale curve of bone within, each one
packaged up like a gift so she had no choice

but to return every evening, at owl light
and wait for that change in the air, the weight
that comes on silent wings, talons trailing
the tips of the wheat, a half-lifetime ago

and still the bleeding, unseen beneath gold,
the skeletons in her pockets, carried home.

Dogs' Balls

So many lost in the long grass of August,
the deep-nettled verges of blowsy lanes.
Perhaps these lush, glimmering weeks
have made us reckless – shedding anoraks
and caution, slinging without judgement or care,
our dogs barking frantic encouragement,
charging before we've drawn back arms –
zig-zagging back, bemused and empty-mouthed.

And if we've misjudged our throws this season,
may we unearth what is ours in the snuffled mulch
by a rain-soaked wall, or be returned to ourselves
in a frozen and leafless park, when a lurcher
arrows through the trees, gently drops
one of summer's perished balls at our feet.

Poem for the Premier Inn

For the carpet, speckled with orange and mauve,
the blackout curtains that don't fully close,
the pale, ribbed shades of the lamps.

For the TV bolted to the mid-beige wall,
the umbilicus fixed to the hairdryer drawer,
the purple-padded headboard and matching throw.

For the sugar-free sweetener, the kettle tray,
the two sachets of *Twining's Everyday*,
the UHT semi-skimmed, the upside-down mugs.

For the canvas of soft-focus lavender heads,
the dog-eared Bible on the chipboard shelf.
For the white hollowfibre pillows,

the wipe-clean signature of Jude
who 'lovingly serviced this room'.
For all those who have stood

at this bolted-down window and gazed
across the car park to the hospital, who stayed,
killing hours until visiting time.

Web on the Wing Mirror

The morning I drove to the hospital
hedges glimmered and a web,

silver-beaded, spanned the wing-mirror,
a spider crouched tight on the edge.

I imagined her, grafting all night –
constructing the scaffolding,

strengthening, testing, tying-off,
suspended like a climber on a rope,

all her energy in this creation,
something of her in every strand.

I could have destroyed her work
with a brush of the hand and yet

I drove so carefully that day –
slowing each time the wind

forced her silk to billow, to bend
and she hung on in there

on a line taut as hope, flickered
like a heartbeat on a twelve-week scan.

Cord

On the fifth day I find it in your cot,
still held firm in a plastic clip.

When the nurse lay you on my chest
it pulsed between us, blue-white

vigorous, the best I had to give –
stem-cell, lymphocytes, streaming

down the line they had to cut off.
Nine months of nurture you shed,

easy as a snake discards its skin
and I'm left holding this wisp of a thing –

a twist of ochre, a garnet swirl,
a swell of black, like a fossilised eye

opaque with remembering.
I hoard it in a matchbox as I would

a seashell, the hook of a cocoon,
a milk tooth, a curl.

Side Effects

After Granddad's death,
my grandma lined up his bottles
and half-empty blister packs
on a windowsill, selected a pill to take
each morning with her cup of tea.
She'd choose another before bed.

Such a cocktail he was given
towards the end – for blood pressure,
heart failure and God-knows-what
but he'd swallow them faithfully,
as stoically as she did now.
Can't let them go to waste she said.

I remember that slight tremor
as she unscrewed tricky lids,
how she'd grasp the backs of chairs
to steady herself up. She never once
claimed to miss him, only that
his tablets had given her that ulcer.

The Dog Who Played with His Shadow

I saw him on the beach, not running
with the other dogs, but bounding back

    and forth, fixated on the moves
    of his darker self, the half-moon quiver

of his tail, the pitch of torso and legs over sand
that bore the slash marks of his claws.

    Abandoned on the moors, his owner said –
    early life unknown, shed and chain at a guess.

Easy to imagine a shiver of wind,
the resulting stutter of light between slats,

    the dart of a paw, how he worried
    himself half to death, scratching out

the only game he knew on a concrete floor,
a compulsion that fed, grew vast

    on small offerings of sun and shade.
    I remember that expanse of shingle and sky,

those seconds of joyous release
before he pinned himself back to the ground.

Clearing
For John

I wake, roll across the bed to where
the mattress still holds your shape.

From outside, the thud and rasp
of a scraper on ice. I picture you, arching
across the bonnet, a plastic handle in your grip,

the expansion of your smoke-signal breath
as you work from outside in –

the windscreen of my car, white-feathered,
blinded by frost and you, prising off
that glittering skin. It's your gloved hands

I'm imagining – the growing warmth
as they clear my vision for the journey ahead.

Acknowledgements

Acknowledgements are due to the editors of the following magazines and anthologies in which versions of some of these poems have appeared: *The North, Mslexia, Poetry Salzburg Review, The River, Fanfare* (Second Light Publications*), The C Word* anthology (Black Cat Poets), *The Heart Pocket Poetry Anthology* (Eye Flash Poetry).

'Pellets' won the Otley Poetry Competition, 2018 under the title of 'Owl Light'; 'Medusa Cuts of Her Snakes' won the PENfro Poetry Competition, 2017; 'The Mechanics of Love' was placed second in the Poetry on the Lake Silver Wyvern Competition, 2017.

I would like to thank the following for their help, support and guidance: Carol Ann Duffy, Ann and Peter Sansom, Gaia Holmes, Sally Baker, Keith Hutson, John Foggin, Sarah Corbett, Simon Zonenblick, Fokkina McDonnell, Marion Oxley and the wonderful Caldergate Poets. Special thanks and love to my family and my husband John.